CAREERS IN

ORTHODONTICS

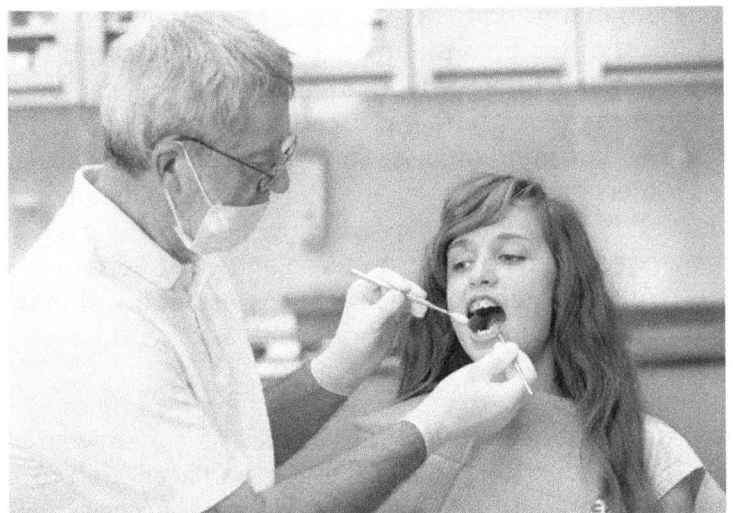

WHAT DO KATY PERRY AND THE high school cheerleader next door have in common? Braces. Braces are dental appliances used to straighten a person's teeth and correct unhealthy overbites or underbites. Braces are usually worn by kids 10 to 14 years old, but many adults wear braces – even celebrities. In fact, of the four million people in the US who wear braces, one million are adults.

Most of the time braces are used for cosmetic reasons.

Everyone wants a beautiful smile, but it is not always a matter of vanity. Crooked teeth and misaligned jaws can cause serious health problems. Teeth that do not fit together right are harder to clean, making the person more at risk for tooth decay, periodontal disease, and even lost teeth. Crooked teeth can also create stress on the jaw and facial muscles that leads to headaches, TMJ syndrome, and pain in the neck, shoulders, or back.

When the need for braces is indicated, the person to see is an orthodontist. An orthodontist is a dentist who specializes in moving teeth and adjusting misaligned jaws. Most of the time that means installing braces, but there are many different types of appliances that can be used to move teeth, retrain muscles, and affect the growth and position of jaws. Some of these devices are fixed, others are removable, and still others are (nearly) invisible. They all work by applying gentle pressure over an extended period of time on teeth and jaws. Some cases require surgery, in which case the orthodontist may perform the surgery or collaborate with another dental specialist.

There is a great need for orthodontists. There are fewer than 10,000 practicing today, which is barely enough to handle the number of people seeking their services. Experts are predicting a job outlook that is better than any other occupation can expect.

Orthodontics is clearly one of the best career choices for long-term job security, but getting started is not easy or fast. It can take more than 10 years of education after graduating from high school. After four years of college earning a bachelor's degree, there is another four years of dental school. Then there is an additional two to three years of specialized training in orthodonture to become eligible for licensing and board certification.

Is the investment in time and money worth it? Practicing orthodontists overwhelmingly say yes and very few ever leave the profession. The most recent US News & World Report ranks orthodontics at #5 among the top 100 jobs in America. The pay is a good basis alone to trumpet this career, with a median salary that is four times what the average worker earns. Other reasons orthodontics came out on top include a great job outlook, low stress level, good work-life balance, and an unemployment rate that is virtually nonexistent.

WHAT YOU CAN DO NOW

START PREPARING FOR THIS CAREER while in high school by loading up on math and science courses. Chemistry, biology, physics, and math are particularly important. Take as many AP science classes as possible to gain college credit hours. Keep your grades up, especially in science courses. When you apply to dental school, heavy emphasis will be placed on your grades in science courses in college. A high GPA in college also gives you the advantage of being eligible for early acceptance programs in some dental schools. Look into that possibility early so you do not miss out.

Orthodontics is a combination of science and art. To develop a good artistic eye, enroll in art classes. A drawing class would be helpful. Sculpture would be even better since you will need experience with modeling or plasters. Hand skills are a basic necessity. Look for ways to develop your manual dexterity, such as playing a musical instrument.

Before making the commitment to years of training, make sure this is the career you truly want. The best way to learn about the field is to job shadow. You can ask your guidance counselor to help you set one up, or you can simply contact a local professional. Shadowing is watching everything the orthodontist does and asking questions. It can give you a general feel for the environment, but really understanding what the work entails requires more time. Try to get a job in an orthodontist's office or volunteer. In addition to learning more about the profession, it will make you a stronger dental school applicant.

Dental schools expect a high GPA, but they also look for involvement in extracurricular activities like volunteer work, community service, or leadership in school organizations and clubs. The best activities are related to dentistry, such as school health careers clubs, dental camps, or volunteering in clinical settings. These provide opportunities to gather valuable letters of recommendation from instructors and supervisors.

Join the American Student Dental Association (ASDA). This organization is dedicated to preparing you for dental school.

HISTORY OF THE CAREER

AS A PROFESSION, ORTHODONTICS has been around for about 100 years. However, humans have always been born with crowded, crooked teeth as well as overbites and other forms of malocclusion that affect the ability to chew and speak. Archaeologists have confirmed this by examining human remains dating back 50,000 years. Since 1000 BC, attempts have been made to correct these problems. Crude metal bands were found around the teeth of Egyptian mummies. It is believed that catgut was used to tie the bands and move the teeth.

Similar primitive attempts at orthodontics were made by the ancient Greeks, Romans, and Etruscans. Greek physician Hippocrates was the first to write about tooth irregularities in 400 BC. Celsus, a Roman writer, suggested a regular regimen of pushing newly emerging teeth with fingers to ensure their proper position. Another Roman writer, Pliny the Elder, recommended filing the longest teeth to match the size of shorter ones.

Orthodontics remained undeveloped until the 17th century, when dental impressions were introduced by German surgeon Matthaeus Gottfried Purmann, who reported using wax to take impressions. About 100 years later, another German surgeon, Phillip Pfaff, used plaster of Paris. More progress was made in the 18th century.

Finally, there was a surge of progress in the 18th century. French physician, Pierre Fauchard, invented an appliance called "bandeau," a piece of metal with spaced holes designed to correct tooth alignment. Fauchard also used a more aggressive technique, using forceps to force teeth into position before tying them in place while they healed. The first complete scientific description of dentistry, written by Fauchard, was published in 1728. It earned him the label, "Father of Dentistry."

Until the early 18th century, the practice of orthodontics was called "regulation." That changed when French dentist, Dr. Lefoulon came up with the term "orthodontisie."

In the US, significant advancements in the field began in the 19th century. Most were focused on correcting poor teeth alignment. A device called the "bite plane" was used to address grinding of misaligned teeth. The appliance later morphed into the Bionator and Herbst devices that are used today. The occipital anchorage, a type of headgear designed to pressure teeth from outside the mouth, was invented in 1822 by J. S. Gunnell. Published in 1841, *The Dental Art,* described techniques such as soldering knobs onto bands and utilizing gold caps to open the dental bite.

Despite the development of various teeth straightening devices, it was common for dentists in the 19th century to extract teeth that were problematic. This practice led to the need for good replacements. In the last decade of the century, orthodontist Edward H. Angle became increasingly interested in dental occlusion and how to treat malocclusion. His work led directly to the development of modern orthodontics as a separate and established profession, which is why he is known as the "Father of Modern Orthodontics." Angle introduced a new system of diagnosing and classifying cases for the most appropriate type of treatment.

Around the same time that Angle was perfecting his scientific system, two books were published on the subject of orthodontics – the first time any publication had been devoted exclusively to the topic. One was *The Significance of the Natural Form and Arrangement of the Dental Arch of Man.* Written by French dentist, I. B. Davenport, it was the first recommendation against the extraction of teeth whenever possible. The other book, written by Dr. Henry Baker, proposed the idea of using elastics or rubber bands to treat malocclusion.

Modern Orthodontics

The field of orthodontics in the 20th century was marked mostly by refinements of previously introduced appliances and treatment methods. For example, until the 1970s, brackets were anchored to teeth by tying wires around each tooth. With the invention of dental adhesives, that basic technique changed to sticking the brackets directly onto tooth surfaces. Gold and silver, which had long been the most common choice for wire, were replaced by stainless steel. The metal was much cheaper, making braces available to more people who might not have been able to afford them before. Lingual braces, which are applied to the inside of teeth surfaces, addressed any aesthetic concerns.

Today's orthodontic treatment has been elevated to a biological art. It is efficient, comfortable, and relatively fast compared to what patients could expect in the past. Many new innovations have come along in just the past two decades that have yielded excellent results. Temporary anchorage devices like Miniscrews have replaced uncomfortable headgear. Self-ligating brackets are not only more comfortable, they result in faster treatment and fewer office visits for archwire changes. Older patients, who typically dislike the aesthetics of metal braces, can substitute clear, removable teeth aligners like Invisaligns. Rather than be limited to the two-dimensional views of X-rays, orthodontists can now use Cone-beam computed tomography (CBCT) to see a patient's jaws and teeth in three dimensions. This 3D imaging helps the practitioner make a more precise diagnosis and treatment plan.

WHERE YOU WILL WORK

MOST ORTHODONTISTS WORK either as a sole practitioner in their own office, or as an associate or partner in a multi-specialty dental office. You can also find them working in the offices of physicians, the offices of other types of health practitioners, general and surgical hospitals, and outpatient care facilities. A small number are in academia, research, or the military.

The vast majority of orthodontists work in private practice as a sole proprietor. They spend the first few years concentrating on growing their client base. Starting out, most patients are referred by other dentists who do not have the same level of specialized training and experience. As time goes on, referrals also come from past clients who were happy with the service they received.

It is rare for an orthodontist to open a practice immediately upon the completion of training. It takes experience and a sizable financial investment to open a practice. The usual route is to take a job, or a series of jobs, as an associate in an established orthodontist's office. After a few years, the associate will be seasoned and ready to become a partner, open a practice, or go a different route altogether, such as surgery or research.

Orthodontists' offices and clinics are bright and nicely furnished. The environment is designed to put nervous patients at ease, but such comfortable working conditions also benefit the practitioners. Most orthodontists, particularly those who run their own practices, are able to control their own schedule and patient load. The result is workweeks that are shorter than those of most healthcare professionals. On average, an orthodontist works about 30 to 40 hours per week. There is rarely overtime, though some adjust their schedules to accommodate patients who work during the day. Being on call is also rare since emergencies are highly unlikely.

THE WORK YOU WILL DO

ORTHODONTICS IS THE AREA OF DENTISTRY that specifically addresses dental irregularities, such as crooked teeth, spacing problems, overbite, and underbite. Orthodontists are trained to diagnose and take corrective measures to straighten teeth and properly align jaws.

The number one reason people go to the orthodontist is to get braces. We have all seen braces, those dental straps or wires that use pressure to correct the teeth structure inside a person's mouth. Sometimes elastic bands are added to help correct jaw movements. Some people go directly to the orthodontist when their teeth are not straight and it bothers them. Others are referred by their general dentist who may notice an improper bite, crowded teeth that are difficult to clean and are destined to become decayed, or complaints of clicking or pain in the jaw.

People of all ages may need and wear braces, but roughly 80 percent of orthodontic patients are kids in their teens. At that age, the teeth and face are still growing so it is the perfect time to intervene with corrective measures. Over an extended period of time, braces can gently guide the teeth into proper alignment, keeping them straight and avoiding future malocclusion issues.

The first step for an orthodontist is to perform a thorough exam. Then, by studying x-rays and plaster models of the teeth, a diagnosis is made. The orthodontist will determine the most appropriate treatment based on the individual's dental irregularities. Any necessary dental appliances are ordered and installed. The patient's progress is monitored for the duration of the treatment period and adjustments are made during regularly scheduled visits. When the desired result has been achieved, the appliances are removed and the patient returns once a year for check-ups.

Orthodontic treatment can take a long time. Most young people who get braces will wear them for two or three years. Some orthodontists specialize in accelerated teeth straightening, a method that is usually reserved for adults. Instead of seeing the orthodontist every six to eight weeks for adjustments, braces are tightened every two weeks. The desired result is typically achieved in six months – a serious benefit for adults who do not want to look like a kid with a mouthful of metal for as short a time as possible. Because an adult's teeth have been heading in the wrong direction for many years, permanent retainers are usually applied to keep them from shifting back into their original position.

Adults who do not want to be seen wearing braces at all can also take advantage of new technology that uses clear plastic mouth retainers such as those made by Invisalign. They are vacuum-formed to the teeth and do not cover the roof of the mouth, so teeth do not shift and speech is not affected. For kids who do not want their braces to show, there are lingual braces. These are braces installed behind the teeth rather than in the front, so they are not easily noticed. Both of these options are comfortable and efficient, but they are also more expensive than traditional methods.

Most people think of orthodontics as a type of cosmetic work. While it is true that the majority of an orthodontist's time is spent straightening teeth and thereby creating beautiful smiles, an orthodontist is capable of much more. They deal with all kinds of conditions including cleft lip, facial abnormalities, skeletal problems, jaw pain, speech impediments, sleep apnea, gum disease, and chewing difficulties. Most of these issues can be dealt with by correcting an overbite or underbite or by altering the shape of the jaw. In some cases, surgery is called for.

Surgery

Some orthodontic treatments require surgery. Depending on the type of surgery required, the orthodontist may perform the surgery or refer the case to an oral surgeon. Orthodontic surgery can provide significant benefits. It can ward off future jaw problems, ensure that treatments have long lasting results, help treat gum conditions, and make it easier to thoroughly clean teeth.

There are several kinds of orthodontic surgery. The most common is tooth extraction. Nobody likes to lose teeth, but sometimes it is necessary to alleviate crowding and bite problems. The teeth most likely to be removed are the wisdom teeth, which are arguably useless anyway.

Another type of common orthodontic surgery is a fiberotomy. This is a procedure that involves detaching the fibers surrounding a tooth. Those fibers are nature's way of holding teeth in place, which can be a problem if you want the teeth to be in a different position. A fiberotomy is usually performed after teeth have been repositioned with braces. It is intended to help the teeth stay in the new position and not naturally drift back to the old position that has been corrected.

The field of orthodontics often overlaps with other dental specialties, such as oral and maxillofacial surgery, orthognathics, or prosthedontics. Oral and maxillofacial surgery addresses the movement of both the teeth and the jawbone. Conditions requiring this type of surgery often involve the combined efforts of both types of surgeons.

Orthognathics is corrective jaw surgery. It is used to correct various problems and conditions of the jaw and face, such as sleep apnea, TMJ disorders, severe malocclusion caused by skeletal misalignment, and congenital conditions like cleft palate. Orthognatics goes hand in hand with orthodontics, but it is different because it deals primarily with bones rather than teeth. Procedures usually involve cutting and realigning bones, and then using screws or plates to hold them in place.

Orthodontic treatment sometimes calls for implants. Implant procedures can be done by an orthodontic surgeon, but they are generally considered the domain of the prosthodontist.

Orthodontic Assistant (OA)

The first person you see at the orthodontist's office after checking in is the assistant. These assistants, or OAs as they are commonly known, prepare the appointment room and do all the preliminary work needed before the orthodontist takes over. This includes cleaning up after the previous patient's visit, sterilizing the orthodontist's equipment, and laying out any hand tools that the orthodontist may need for the next appointment.

On the first visit, the OA will meet the new patient and discuss the issues that need to be addressed. The OA will take an oral history and conduct a preliminary examination. Depending on the level of skills and experience, an OA may also take X-rays and photographs of the mouth and make impressions of the patient's teeth. During the visit, the OA hands the necessary tools to the orthodontist during the examination and treatment. At the end of the visit, the OA gives instructions to patients on how to care for any devices and how to clean appliances in their mouth.

At subsequent visits, the OA prepares the patient for the orthodontist by conducting a preliminary examination, discussing any problems or concerns, tightening braces, and changing out wires and brackets if required.

In smaller practices, the orthodontic assistant may also perform administrative duties, including setting appointments, billing, writing up charts, and maintaining patient records. It is common for OAs to do lab work as well, such as pouring and trimming patient molds.

The job of an OA is very different than that of a dental assistant. Dental assistants rarely see the patient without the dentist being present. Their responsibility is to stand by the dentist's side during procedures, passing instruments and operating the suction equipment. Orthodontic assistants are more independent. They actually spend more time working alone with the patient than they do assisting the orthodontist. In most cases, they are free to use their own judgment as to what tasks should be done.

ORTHODONTISTS TELL ABOUT THEIR CAREERS

I Am an Associate Orthodontist

"Being an associate simply means working for another orthodontist rather than having my own practice. I work under contract with a base salary, plus monthly bonuses based on the number of patients I treat. I've worked as an associate for three other employers, but my current situation is the best so far.

I think most orthodontists go into the field for the same reason I did. I had crooked teeth and an overbite as a kid that really affected how I felt about myself. After orthodontics, I felt completely different, full of confidence. I wanted to give that same experience to other kids, so becoming an orthodontist was an obvious career choice for me. Today, when I look at the before and after pictures of my young patients, I am still amazed at the difference. Seeing their smiles when the job is done is the most wonderful part of my job.

This is rewarding work, but it can also be quite challenging. I typically see at least 50 patients a day. Most of them are scheduled in the afternoon when they get out of school. These are quick visits that usually take less than 10 minutes to change wires or tighten braces. Things that take longer, like installing new braces, are done in the morning. Occasionally, there are tough cases that require surgery or teaming up with other healthcare professionals.

I have the opportunity to develop meaningful relationships with patients over the span of a few years. That can be very gratifying and sometimes surprising, especially with kids. I don't know if they think I'm a therapist or a big brother, but I hear it all – sibling rivalry issues, the hatred of math homework, who likes who this week, and on and on. I listen intently and laugh later when they're gone.

My advice to anyone who is thinking of orthodontics as a career is to make sure it's what you really want before you commit. Contact as many practitioners as you can and pick their brains. Shadow at least one or two for a full day. Read trade publications and scour the internet for news about advancements in the field. It will take many years of hard work to become an established orthodontist, but if the work suits you, it will be worth it."

I Am an Orthodontist's Assistant

"After the front desk, I am the first person you will meet at this orthodontist's office. People are often surprised by how much I do before they see the orthodontist. When I meet a new patient, I spend a couple of minutes chatting to put them at ease. Then I take x-rays and photographs of their mouth, and take impressions of their teeth. I also see existing patients before the orthodontist. Depending on where they are in the procedure, I might polish and prepare their teeth before braces are installed. My orthodontist has me help apply the braces, but not all assistants do that. After braces are on, I finish attaching the wires and teach the patients how to clean their teeth. On subsequent visits, I conduct a preliminary examination and simply tighten the braces.

My job is very different than that of a dental assistant. Anyone who has been to a family dentist knows what the dental assistant does – sits next to the dentist, passes instruments and operates the irrigation and suction equipment. You always see assistants in the presence of the dentist. My work is much more independent. That's one of the best things about my job. I even have my own office, which dental assistants don't. An orthodontic assistant's responsibilities can be quite extensive, too. For example, if there is a lab on site, they might make molds, mouthguards, or retainers.

There is a lot to like about this career. It's flexible. I could choose to work part time, which a lot of orthodontic assistants do. I prefer to work full time,

40 hours a week. It's stable. I never work overtime or on weekends. General dentistry offices often run late, but that is not the case in orthodontics. We rarely run into unexpected complications that would push appointments back.

There are plenty of job opportunities and the pay is good considering the training required."

I Am a Sole Practitioner With My Own Practice

"I have a medium sized practice in a medium sized city. It's a general practice that serves patients of all ages, but kids account for about 80 percent. You have to enjoy kids to be an orthodontist, and I do. I like hearing about their day and what's going on in the schools. I really get to know them and their families, especially when there are several siblings to treat over the years. Adults are fun to treat, too, but they're different. Instead of telling me about their lives, they want to know about what I'm doing. I'm happy to show them and explain the physics behind the treatment. They appreciate being informed about what's been done and what to expect next.

Orthodontics is challenging work that keeps me busy and alert. The basic tools and appliances are always the same, but no two people are alike. Every day there are new patients walking in the door and with them comes something new and different to think about. The only thing I know for sure is no two people will require the exact same treatment. In order to make sure I'm doing what is best for my patients, I meet regularly with a group of dentists here in town. We call it a study group and it is much like the study groups I remember from college. It is a very important part of my practice because it provides a chance to learn from other kinds of dentistry specialists. The more I know about all areas of dentistry, the better orthodontist I can be.

Most orthodontic students look forward to having their own practices. It certainly offers benefits over being a salaried employee, like freedom, flexibility, and greater income potential. You have to keep in mind that it's a business, one that happens to involve straightening teeth. It takes several hours a week just to take care of non-dentistry tasks like paying bills and reviewing state compliance laws. Still, orthodontics is a rewarding profession that offers opportunities to serve the community."

PERSONAL QUALIFICATIONS

BEING AN ORTHODONTIST REQUIRES A UNIQUE combination of skills, including commitment to long-term goals, endless energy, creativity, a knack for fixing things, and a head for science. If you think you are up to the challenge, here are some more traits that will help you become successful in the field.

Excellent communications skills are essential. Throughout the day, orthodontists talk with patients and their families, teaching them how to care for their teeth while wearing braces and what to expect until the next visit. They also routinely communicate with orthodontic assistants and lab technicians. It is important that they give clear instructions to their assistants and just as important that they listen to what the assistants tell them about the patients.

Are you a people person? Orthodontists work closely with patients over long periods of time, often several years. During that time, they must always present a positive outlook and alleviate any fears. They work with people of all ages, but they usually treat mostly children and teens. This can be a challenge since kids can require patience. A sense of humor definitely helps.

Orthodontics is equally mental and physical. Years of education that focus on the natural sciences provide the necessary intellectual skills, but it takes physical stamina to do this work since you will be bending over patients for long periods. Manual dexterity is also necessary. The very nature of orthodontics requires spending time working with your hands in confined spaces in the mouth. If you are good with your hands, you will be able to master the many specialized tools to do the work well.

Small details matter in orthodontics. Orthodontists must pay close attention to the shape and size of each tooth, as well the relationship to teeth above, below, and adjoining. Adjustments to braces are done in very small increments. Too much movement can cause pain and other problems.

Orthodontics is all about solving problems. Successful orthodontists enjoy fixing things and figuring out long-term solutions.

ATTRACTIVE FEATURES

IT TAKES MANY YEARS OF EDUCATION and training to become an orthodontist. Following through on such a major commitment requires dedication and the hope that it will all be worth it. US News & World Report offers some very good news for those who may have doubts. In its most recent yearly survey, orthodontics was ranked #5 among the top 100 jobs in America based on employment rate, salary, 10-year job outlook, stress level, and work-life balance. At the top of the list was dentistry, but orthodontics has a median salary that is $35,000 a year more than general dentistry. The average orthodontist also makes about four times more than the average worker across all occupations. Dentistry only came out on top in one category – more total job openings than orthodontics.

Orthodontics promises great prospects for rapid job growth over the coming decade. It is a field with virtually no unemployment. This level of job security is unheard of in most industries. Too few new orthodontists are graduating to treat the growing patient population, but the main reason for the low unemployment rate is those in the profession rarely leave before retirement. Most find the work enjoyable and fulfilling, both professionally and personally.

Orthodontics is satisfying because it helps people feel better about themselves. It does not offer instant gratification – it usually takes several years for a patient to complete the process. During that time the relationship between orthodontist and patient grows stronger as the patient becomes more confident and the orthodontist sees gradual changes that portend a great result. In the end, a beautiful smile and a grateful patient are tremendously satisfying rewards.

It may seem that an orthodontist has few options, but actually there is a wide range of career opportunities. You can be a solo practitioner or enter a partnership with one or more colleagues. Some orthodontists dedicate their career to research and teaching. Those with an altruistic bent work with public health agencies or the military. Patients are typically children or teenagers, but some orthodontists specialize in treating adults.

This is also a field that lets you choose where and how you want to work and live. Pick any location and you can probably practice there. If you want the freedom to enjoy life outside of the office, you can do that. Work schedules are flexible. A workweek of only three or four days is common and overtime is rare. Solo practitioners are essentially free to pursue their own priorities.

For those who do not want to spend many years in school, becoming an orthodontist assistant is a good alternative. There are minimal education requirements to prepare for the career. It typically takes one year to complete a certificate program that qualifies beginners for entry-level positions working alongside orthodontists. Once qualified, the job prospects are excellent, on a par with orthodontists. The hours are good. Not only is overtime uncommon, but there is often a choice of part-time or full-time work. Finally, orthodontist assistants have autonomy. Unlike dentist assistants, these professionals conduct most of their work independently without anyone looking over their shoulder.

UNATTRACTIVE ASPECTS

AS REWARDING AND LUCRATIVE AS A CAREER in orthodontics can be, the path is not an easy one. Despite the obvious advantages of pursuing this specialty, the American Association of Orthodontists reports that only six out of 100 dental school graduates continues on to become orthodontists. Although this career pays more than general dentistry, the additional education can be challenging. After spending eight to 10 years in college and dentistry school, another three years of advanced orthodontic training are required for certification. This is not only a big investment in time, there are costs to consider. It is not surprising that most dental school graduates would rather start practicing and start repaying student loans.

Beyond the educational requirements, there is not much to dislike about the career. There is very little stress associated with the work. Occasionally, an orthodontist must face an unhappy patient or parent of a child whose years of treatment did not meet their expectations. This is the exception rather than the rule, however.

Orthodontic procedures can also cause pain. A good orthodontist continually commiserates and reassures patients that the final results will be worth any discomfort. Some orthodontists do not like spending their days working in patients' mouths, but that does not seem to stop most from continuing in the field.

Orthodontist assistants do not face the same educational challenges as orthodontists. However, advancement opportunities are very limited without more education.

EDUCATION AND TRAINING

PROSPECTIVE ORTHODONTISTS should be prepared to spend many years in school. The basic requirement is a doctorate degree in dentistry followed by specialized training in orthodontics. On average, that takes 11 years.

The path usually starts in college, earning a bachelor's degree. Technically, a degree is not required to get into dental school as long as the student has taken the prerequisite courses such as organic chemistry and physiology, and passed with high grades. It is unlikely, however, that any student would be sufficiently prepared for the rigors of dental school without completing four years of college.

Bachelor's Degree

College for prospective orthodontists is all about preparing for dental school. There is no particular major required for admission to dental school, but a major in science is certainly the most useful. Regardless of the major, there will be some pre-dental courses included in your curriculum, such as biology, physics, chemistry, and a few others.

It is extremely important to maintain a good GPA, especially for all of the prerequisite classes required by dental school. Without high grades in these classes, admission is unlikely. Undergraduate students should also develop excellent study habits and learn to focus when classes and work get difficult.

In addition to high GPA scores, dental schools will require Dental Aptitude Test (DAT) scores. Minimum DAT score requirements vary among dental schools, but schools are selective and only students with high scores have a chance of admission. The multiple-choice test covers reading comprehension, math skills, and quantitative reasoning. It is designed to demonstrate that the student has the knowledge and critical thinking skills that will be needed for the difficult courses ahead.

Dental School

Dental school involves four years of intense study that includes both classroom instruction and clinical training. The first two years are focused on scientific coursework such as physiology, microbiology, biochemistry, and anatomy. The classes are very rigorous, going into great depth and detail about various systems of the body that may be affected by the work of a dentist.

The last two years are dedicated to clinical work. During this time, students learn the basic skills a dentist needs, including performing a dental exam, cleaning teeth, filling cavities, tooth extractions, and treating gum disease. They master their skills under the direct supervision of licensed dentists. By the time they are finished, they are able to handle every procedure a patient may require. Upon graduation, they are awarded a Doctor of Dental Medicine degree.

Orthodontics Postgraduate Training

After finishing dental school, most graduates are ready to start their careers as dentists. Those who intend to practice orthodontics, however, must continue their training. Fewer than 10 percent of dental school graduates pursue this additional specialized training. Acceptance is highly competitive and very selective.

Orthodontic programs accredited by the American Dental

Association can last anywhere from two to five years. Clearly, only the most dedicated individuals are up for the challenge. The programs provide in-depth courses in biomedical, behavioral, and basic sciences. The focus is on the development of the skills needed to facilitate tooth movement, guide facial changes, and understand facial surgery. Orthodontists are also trained to diagnose and treat other problems related to the face and neck.

Licensure and Certification

Orthodontists must be licensed in order to practice. Licensing requirements vary from state to state, but generally include graduation from an established school and completing a postgraduate program in orthodontics. In many states, a license allows the practice of orthodontics and general dentistry.

Certification is not a legal requirement for the practice of orthodontics, but it is highly recommended because it helps demonstrate a high level of proficiency to employers and patients. Board certification is available through the American Board of Orthodontics. To earn it, candidates must pass a very thorough exam. The written portion covers 27 different subjects, while the clinical part involves evaluating an entire set of case records for which the candidate must develop treatment plans.

Orthodontist Assistant

Some states consider orthodontic assistants to be the same as dental assistants. Other states recognize that OAs have expanded roles that require specialized training. In either case, there are two levels of training: certificate programs and associate degrees. Some community colleges and vocational schools offer courses in orthodontic assisting. Most only offer dental assisting programs with the opportunity to work for an orthodontist who will oversee the clinical side of the program. The end result is roughly the same.

Admission requirements usually include a high school diploma or GED plus CPR certification. It typically takes one year to complete a program that includes 52 hours of classroom instruction and 500 hours working in an orthodontic practice. Upon completion, students are awarded a certificate that qualifies them for assistant positions.

The more ambitious route for prospective orthodontist assistants is to pursue an associate degree in dental assisting. These are two-year programs offered through community colleges that include general education courses plus clinical and technical training. Students are usually required to complete internships or externships in a dental clinic.

EARNINGS

ORTHODONTISTS ARE AMONG THE HIGHEST PAID professionals in any field. Orthodontics is typically ranked in the top 20 highest-paid occupations in the US with an average annual salary of $225,000. Even the lowest paid orthodontists – who are usually those new to the profession – average more than $100,000. Only those who are still in training earn less.

The highest paid orthodontists are those with the most experience. Those seasoned professionals can earn upwards of $500,000 a year. The actual income of any orthodontist depends on various factors, including number of years on the job, number of patients, type of employer, and location.

Experience is the key factor in this field. Regardless of where an orthodontist works or what type of organization is hiring, experience will influence the overall earnings more than anything else. Experienced orthodontists are highly valued partly for their skills, but also because they have learned how to put new patients at ease and gain their trust. Experience is also important because with every passing year, an established orthodontist's patient list grows. The earnings of an orthodontist are directly related to the number of patients being treated. As their reputation spreads, more and more referrals come in until, at some point, the practice is at full capacity – the ultimate goal of any professional.

The type of employer also impacts an orthodontist's income. Most orthodontists work in private practice, as part of a dental group, or in hospitals. Other dentists offer the most jobs. Orthodontists who work in the offices of other dentists earn an average salary of nearly $210,000 with the opportunity to earn much more if they grow their patient list. A small number of orthodontists work for other health professionals, earning around $185,000 annually.

Orthodontists who operate their own private practices earn far more than their salaried colleagues. A successful practice can net profits of $400,000 to more than $600,000. That is after overhead, but before self-paid benefits such as health insurance and retirement plans. Independent orthodontists who are part of a dental group or partnership may receive ownership benefits. Typically, this is based on a percentage of annual net profits. In some cases, it is based on the overall number of patients.

The lowest salaries are paid to those employed by hospitals. Private hospitals pay more than state hospitals. Annual earnings average about $125,000 in private hospitals, while state facilities pay around $100,000. Outpatient care centers offer an average of $170,000.

Regardless of the type of employer, the size of the employer is a determining factor. The size is directly proportional to the number of patients. Generally, a larger establishment has a greater chance of building a good reputation that attracts new patients.

Geographic location can also make a big difference in pay. Unlike many professionals, orthodontists do better in smaller towns and rural areas than in big cities. This is due to the level of competition. There are more orthodontists per capita in highly populated urban areas, which forces each to lower their prices in order to attract new patients. In less populated areas, there is usually only one orthodontist within miles around. Such exclusivity makes it possible to set prices without the concern that someone else will offer lower fees. The cost of living and especially the cost of doing business should also be considered. Office space in New York can be 10 times more than the same space in Kentucky.

The states with the highest average earnings for orthodontists are Tennessee, Georgia, South Carolina, Minnesota, Michigan, and Wisconsin. Those in Texas, Oklahoma, Kentucky, Kansas, Virginia, and Pennsylvania, also do well with average salaries ranging between $235,000 and $250,000. That is about the same as the highest-paying jobs in New York City where the cost of living is extremely high.

Orthodontic Assistants

The earnings of orthodontic assistants are very good for an easy entry field. The median income is about $35,000, but that usually is not a salary. Most assistants are paid hourly wages. Because they work an average 30 hours per week, it is important to take this into consideration when determining what your income might be. A median income of $32,000, for example, works out to $21 per hour for 30 hours a week.

Benefits

Salaried orthodontists also receive a number of benefits that add to the overall compensation. All benefits packages include health insurance and paid time off for vacation and sick days. Retirement benefits are also routinely included. Depending on the type of employer, they are commonly enrolled in a retirement plan. Some employers offer matching contributions to those plans. Orthodontists may also receive year-end bonuses based on the number of patients they treat. Orthodontists in private practice are responsible for their own insurance and benefits.

OPPORTUNITIES

ORTHODONTICS IS A GROWING PROFESSION. It is the largest group of dental specialists in the US, and the number of orthodontists is rapidly increasing. There are more than 9,700 orthodontists practicing today and experts predict another 1,500 positions to open up over the coming decade. That growth rate is faster than the rate of most other occupations, making orthodontics one of the best career choices for long-term job security.

Many positions will open up as older generations of orthodontists retire, but the rosy job outlook is primarily due to an increasing desire for specialized dental care. Over the past few decades, there has been a growing popular trend in the US for cosmetic procedures of all kinds. Since teeth are particularly noticeable, there is no shortage of work for orthodontists. People want to look good, and many are able pay for it.

Advances are made in the field of orthodontics all the time. Continuing education is a must in order to stay up to date with the latest techniques and technology. Those professionals who do stay current are the most likely to successfully compete for open job positions and new patients.

GETTING STARTED

YOU SHOULD BEGIN YOUR JOB SEARCH during your postgraduate training. Start by deciding where you want to live. Keep in mind that the best opportunities for both job openings and income potential are in less populated areas. It can be harder to get started in big cities because of the competition. Of course, if you want to be close to family and friends, your decision is already made.

Occasionally, an internship or residency can turn into a permanent full-time position. This is not something you can count on. You should assume you will be starting fresh somewhere else. The two main ways orthodontists find jobs are through networking and direct contact.

Start networking as early as possible. Contacts and referrals can come from anywhere. Even high school teachers and your own dentist could lead you to a job opportunity. Call them, reintroduce yourself, and ask if they know anyone looking to hire an associate. Other possibilities include college professors and contacts made through volunteering or part-time jobs. The most valuable networking opportunities, however, will come while you are in training. You will need to be assertive and ask for referrals. Gather as many contacts as possible, with or without referrals in mind. When you do get a referral, be sure to ask for permission to use the contact's name. It is always best to have a name to get your foot in the door for an interview.

Be creative. Who else knows of openings before the general public? Supply reps for dental supply companies know all the dentists and orthodontists in the area. In fact, they often keep track of which offices are getting ready to hire. To find these supply reps, call any dentist and ask who services their practice. Another good source is members of your local dental organization. It is very likely they provide placement services.

Once you have exhausted all logical options that involve actually speaking with people, it is time to go online. Begin your search with job sites that are dedicated to dental or medical specialties, such as IHireDental.com. The ADA Career Center is a great online resource for searching for orthodontist positions anywhere in the country. Next, check LinkedIn. It is a snap to search for the type of job you want within the particular area you want. Make sure you have a polished profile completed before you make any contacts through LinkedIn. Finally, turn to the general job sites, Indeed and GlassDoor. These sites provide useful information in addition to job listings.

For example, GlassDoor currently lists hundreds of jobs for orthodontists, with an average salary of over $240,000.

ASSOCIATIONS

■ **American Association of Orthodontists**
https://www.aaoinfo.org

■ **World Federation of Orthodontists**
http://www.wfo.org

■ **International Association for Orthodontics**
https://www.iaortho.org

■ **American Orthodontic Society**
http://www.orthodontics.com

■ **Health Occupations Students of America (HOSA)**
http://www.hosa.org

■ **American Student Dental Association (ASDA)**
https://www.asdanet.org/

PERIODICALS

■ **American Journal of Orthodontics & Dentofacial Orthopedics**
http://www.ajodo.org

■ **The Angle Orthodontist**
http://www.angle.org

■ **Journal of Clinical Orthodontics**
https://www.jco-online.com

www.ingramcontent.com/pod-product-compliance
Lightning Source LLC
Chambersburg PA
CBHW070522220526
45467CB00002B/801